Aline Valéria Martins Pereira

Overweight and food consumption

Aline Valéria Martins Pereira

Overweight and food consumption

Their association in preschoolers at a public day-care center in Rio das Ostras

ScienciaScripts

Imprint
Any brand names and product names mentioned in this book are subject to trademark, brand or patent protection and are trademarks or registered trademarks of their respective holders. The use of brand names, product names, common names, trade names, product descriptions etc. even without a particular marking in this work is in no way to be construed to mean that such names may be regarded as unrestricted in respect of trademark and brand protection legislation and could thus be used by anyone.

Cover image: www.ingimage.com

This book is a translation from the original published under ISBN 978-613-9-65474-1.

Publisher:
Sciencia Scripts
is a trademark of
Dodo Books Indian Ocean Ltd. and OmniScriptum S.R.L publishing group

120 High Road, East Finchley, London, N2 9ED, United Kingdom
Str. Armeneasca 28/1, office 1, Chisinau MD-2012, Republic of Moldova, Europe
Printed at: see last page
ISBN: 978-620-7-77763-1

SUMMARY

SUMMARY

With the increasing participation of women in the job market, there is a need for institutions where mothers can leave their children while they are away from home. This role is fulfilled by nurseries and nursery schools, which are also responsible for feeding the children while they are there. These places have a great responsibility for the nutritional status of these children, which is why this study aimed to investigate the prevalence of overweight and its association with food consumption in children at a public nursery school in the municipality of Rio das Ostras. The children analyzed in this study had their body mass and height/length measured in order to obtain their BMI (Body Mass Index), which was applied to the WHO growth curves (2006-2007) and classified according to the parameters established by the WHO (2006) using the WHO ANTHRO program, and parents and/or guardians were also given a questionnaire on food consumption and socioeconomic status.

1. INTRODUCTION

According to the Law of Guidelines and Bases of National Education (LDBEN), nurseries are institutions that cater for children from zero to three years old, as well as pre-schools, from four to six years old. These two age groups comprise early childhood education, the first stage of basic education, whose purpose is the integral development of the child in its physical, psychological, intellectual and social aspects (BRASIL, 1996).

Day care is a significant need of the population, as a result of the socio-economic transformations that society is undergoing. Children spend eight to ten hours a day in daycare and, during this time, they receive two-thirds of the nutritional recommendation for each age. Therefore, in addition to psycho-pedagogical guidance, it is essential that the food and care offered satisfy their needs and favorably influence their nutritional status (VITOLO, 2008).

Nutritional status is the result of several factors, so the influence of the environment is important. Constant nutritional surveillance is necessary in developing countries due to the high prevalence of disorders such as malnutrition and, more recently, obesity (FILHO & RISSIN, 2003; GUIMARÂES *et al.*, 2001).

Therefore, assessing nutritional status is a fundamental stage in the study of a child, in order to check whether growth is deviating from the expected standard due to some disease and/or unfavorable social conditions. Nutritionally, the period between weaning and the age of five is the most vulnerable phase of a child's life (BRASIL, 2012).

The aim of this study was to investigate the prevalence of overweight and its association with food consumption in children at a public nursery school in the municipality of Rio das Ostras.

2. BACKGROUND

This work is justified by the increase in the number of overweight children in Brazil and, above all, by the risks associated with this condition, such as greater vulnerability to the development of *diabetes mellitus*, dyslipidemia and hypertension. In this sense, the data to be investigated seeks to understand the nutritional status of children, as well as its association with food consumption. These data are important not only for those responsible, but also for health professionals, as they can facilitate the implementation of interventions that minimize the prevalence of excess weight in children, protecting their health.

3. Theoretical framework

The simplest method for knowing nutritional status is anthropometric assessment, which measures variations in physical dimensions and the overall composition of the human body at different ages, and is also used to plan health promotion actions, prevent diseases and carry out early treatment (POLLA & SCHERER, 2011).

As the first years of life are decisive for children's growth and development, monitoring nutritional status at this stage provides relevant information for assessing health and the risks of morbidity and mortality (BRASIL, 2011).

According to the World Health Organization (WORLD HEALTH ORGANIZATION, 2006), sedentary lifestyles and obesity are growing at an alarming rate all over the world, and are no longer merely an aesthetic concern, but a global epidemic.

With regard to the diet of Brazilians, the 2008-2009 Family Budget Survey (POF) revealed an increase in the consumption of food outside the home, a reduction in the consumption of rice, beans, fruit and vegetables and an increase in the consumption of industrialized foods and sugar. As a result, the prevalence of overweight in children aged between five and nine was 25% to 30% in the North and Northeast regions and 32% to 40% in the Southeast, South and Midwest regions (BRASIL, 2009).

The most widely used way of determining obesity is the body mass index (BMI). This anthropometric measure is an indicator that facilitates the verification of excess weight, since it uses only two variables (body mass and height), and is an inexpensive, non-invasive method that is therefore well accepted worldwide (WHO, 1995; BRASIL, 2012).

The use of anthropometric indices has been considered a valid strategy for generating sensitive indicators of nutritional status, particularly during the pre-school years, as they reflect nutritional conditions and, indirectly, the influences of the socio-economic environment (ABRANTES, Marcelo M., LAMOUNIER Joel A.,

COLOSIMO, enrico A., 2002).

According to the main population surveys conducted in the country, there has been a significant reduction in child malnutrition rates and a more significant occurrence of overweight and obesity. Among children under the age of five assessed in the National Demographic and Health Surveys - PNDS, carried out in 1996 and 2006, the prevalence of malnutrition was reduced by around 50%, from 13.5% in the first survey to 6.8% in the most recent one (MONTEIRO & CASTRO, 2009; POLLA; SCHERER, 2011).

The recording of body mass and length, as well as the child's cephalic perimeter, is recommended for all consultations, for children at risk or not, up to the age of two (PANPANICH; GARNER, 2008). Between the ages of two and ten, body mass and height should be measured and recorded on the charts in the Child Health Handbook (BRASIL, 2009).

Among the indices, height-for-age (H/A) deserves to be highlighted, as it best indicates the cumulative effect of adverse situations on a child's growth. It is considered the most sensitive indicator for gauging a population's quality of life (BRASIL, 2011; BRASIL, 2012).

In turn, BMI is used to identify excess weight among children. It is a good marker of adiposity and overweight, as well as being a predictive indicator of BMI in adulthood (BRASIL, 2011).

Several factors influence the genesis of obesity, such as genetic, physiological and metabolic; however, it can be explained that this growing increase in obese individuals seems to be more related to changes in lifestyle and eating habits. The increase in the consumption of foods rich in simple sugars and fat with a high energy density and the decrease in physical exercise are the main factors related to the environment (POLLA; SCHERER, 2011; VITOLO, 2008).

These nutritional imbalances can cause long-term metabolic abnormalities, making students more vulnerable to diseases resulting from inadequate nutrition

(FERNANDES *et al.*, 2012).

In this sense, it is understood that nutritional education is fundamental for health promotion and, for this reason, it must be part of an official national education plan (BIZZO & LEDER, 2005). The Health at School Program (PSE), an intersectoral health and education policy aimed at children, adolescents, young people and adults in Brazilian public education, was set up in 2007 to promote health and comprehensive education (BRASIL, 2009). The link between the school and the basic health network is the basis of the PSE and its strategy is to integrate health and education in order to develop citizenship and qualify Brazilian public policies (BRASIL, 2009).

4. Objectives

The general objective is to investigate the prevalence of overweight and its association with food consumption in children at a public day-care center in the state of São Paulo.

Specifically, the aim is to evaluate the body mass and height of children in a public daycare center in the municipality of Rio das Ostras, as well as to determine the prevalence of overweight in children in a public daycare center in the municipality.

5. METHODS

This is a cross-sectional, descriptive study (Hennekens & Buring, 1987).

5.1 Research subjects

All children between the ages of 8 and 48 months, of both sexes, enrolled in a municipal nursery school located in the Nova Cidade district of Rio das Ostras, R.J., selected for convenience, were invited to take part in this study.

5.2 Ethical considerations

This research was evaluated by the Research Ethics Committee of the Estâcio de Sà University.

All the parents and/or guardians of the children involved in this data collection agreed to take part in this study by signing the Informed Consent Form (ICF) (Appendix 1), after clarifying the objectives and procedures of the research, in accordance with the rules of the National Health Council (Resolution No. 466/2012). The document consists of two pages, each of which must be signed by the parents and/or guardians. Participation in the research was voluntary and participants were informed that there was no remuneration or direct benefits.

As this was an evaluation of children aged between 8 and 48 months, we decided not to ask the participants for their consent.

5.3 Data collection

The municipality of Rio das Ostras - R.J. - has four public kindergartens. The Valdira Flausino Rodrigues nursery school was chosen for convenience. In order to carry out this research, formal permission was requested, by means of a letter of authorization, from the Education Department of the Municipality of Rio das Ostras.

Data was collected in December 2014. The children were identified (name, date of birth and gender) using the enrollment lists obtained from the school office. Prior to data collection, all parents and/or guardians were invited to attend a meeting where the objectives and procedures for data collection were presented. At the end of this meeting, parents and/or guardians were asked to formally authorize the study by signing an Informed Consent Form.

At this point, the parents and/or guardians of the students were invited to complete a questionnaire on food consumption and socioeconomic status (appendices 2 and 3).

A second day of data collection was scheduled, when the children's body mass and height were assessed.

5.4 Anthropometric data collection

The anthropometric measurements were taken in the school environment by the nutrition and nursing teams of the Health at School Program of the Municipal Health and Education Departments of Rio das Ostras, with the support of the teachers and school agents of the above-mentioned nursery school. The data collected was tabulated using the Excel 7.0 program (Microsoft), as shown in Table 1 and, for analysis of the nutritional assessment, the WHO ANTHRO program (World Health Organization Anthro) version 3.2.2 was used (Table 1) and, for a better understanding of the results obtained, tables and graphs were drawn up.

TABLE 1- Spreadsheet used to obtain data on preschoolers.

ID	School Name	Student's name	Class	Valuation Date (D/M/A)	Date of Birth (D/M/A)	Gender M/F	Weight (Kg)	Height (cm)
1								
2								
3								
4								
5								
6								
7								
8								
9								
10								

FIGURE 1- Who Anthro program used for nutritional diagnosis

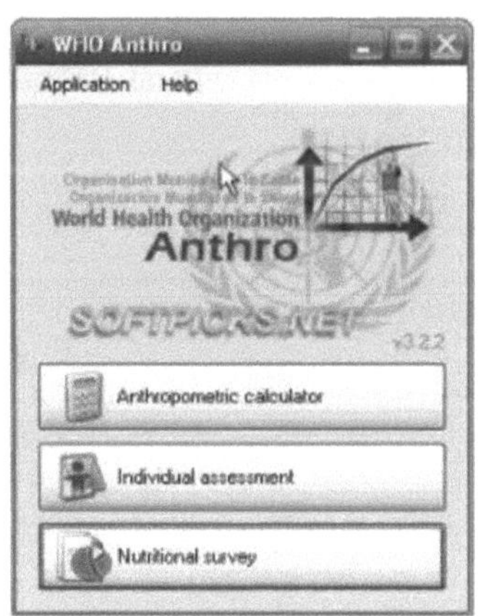

To obtain the children's height/length, an INDAIA BENGALAS infantometer was used, with a maximum measurement of 1 cm and a 0.1 cm scale. Length was measured with the baby lying on a flat surface, upright, with arms stretched out along the body.

For children over 1 meter, a tape measure and a WISO portable stadiometer were used. The tape was attached to a wall, without a corner and in contact with an even floor. The children were positioned upright, motionless, with their arms extended along their bodies and their heads in the *Frankfurt* plane. The back of the neck, shoulders, buttocks and heels remained against the center of the tape, with the knees together. The girls kept their hair loose and unadorned at the time of measurement.

The weight of children under 24 months of age was measured on a WELMY mechanical baby scale with a maximum capacity of 16 kg and a 0.01 kg scale. Children over 24 months were weighed on a LiDER BALANÇAS digital portable scale. The students were weighed wearing as little clothing as possible.

All measurements followed the techniques established by Lohman (1988). The students also had their BMI estimated (body mass/stature^2) and, once this index had been obtained, it was analyzed according to gender, age and height.

For the classification of nutritional status, the child growth curves and their cut-off points established by the World Health Organization were used as a reference, as well as the monitoring criteria used by the Ministry of Health through the Food and Nutrition Surveillance System - SISVAN, using the height/age (H/A) and BMI/age (BMI/A) indices, expressed in Z-score values (BRASIL, 2011).

TABLE 2- BMI cut-off points for age for children (0 to 5 years)[1]

CRITICAL VALUES	NUTRITIONAL DIAGNOSIS
< z-score -3	MARKED THINNESS
> z-score -3 and < z-score -2	THINNESS
> z-score -2 and < z-score +1	EUTROPHY
> z-score +1 and <z-score +2	RISK OF OVERWEIGHT
z-score +2 and <z-score +3	OVERWEIGHT
> Z-score +3	OBESITY

Sources: (WHO, 1995), (BRASIL, 2002), (BRASIL, 2005).

TABLE 3- Height-for-age cut-off points for children (0 to 10 years)

CRITICAL VALUES	NUTRITIONAL DIAGNOSIS
< SCORE- Z -3	VERY LOW FOR AGE
>Z-SCORE -3 AND <Z-SCORE -2	LOW HEIGHT FOR AGE
>ESCORE-Z -2	STATURE APPROPRIATE FOR AGE

Sources: (WHO, 1995), (BRASIL, 2002).

After consolidating the data and the nutritional diagnosis, the PSE nutritionists held a meeting with the parents and the school board, with guidance and referrals for consultations with nutritionists at the Basic Health Unit closest to the homes of the overweight and obese students, as shown in the adapted reference and counter-reference document in Annex 3.

1 Note: The World Health Organization presents weight-for-height references only for children under 5 years of age according to the 2006 growth standard. From this age onwards, the Body Mass Index for age should be used to assess the proportion between the child's weight and height.

Socio-economic data was collected by applying a structured questionnaire to the parents and/or guardians, containing the following variables: name and age of mother and child, gender of the child, whether they have other children and how many, marital status, parents and/or guardians' schooling, who they currently live with, how many people live in their home, monthly family income, number of people who contribute to the family's income.

To assess the frequency of food consumption, the SISVAN Food Frequency Questionnaire (FFQ) was administered to parents and/or guardians. The questionnaire is divided into food consumption marker forms for children under six months, between six months and less than two years and between two years and less than five years and five years and over. The proposed instrument is specific for recording in the SISVAN computerized system, which is shown in Annex 4. However, it was adapted for the research target group, as there were no children under six months old in the nursery school.

The questions for children between six months and less than two years of age aim to characterize the introduction of food, which should take place from the age of six months. On the other hand, the questions for children between two years and less than five years old, who should have already adopted the family diet, should assess feeding practices at this stage of life (SISVAN/MS-2008).

6. CHARACTERISTICS OF RIO DAS OSTRAS CHILDREN AND THE FOOD THE STUDENTS EAT

School meals in Brazil have been guaranteed since 1955 by the National School Feeding Program (PNAE), which guarantees, through the transfer of financial resources by the National Education Development Fund (FNDE), the feeding of all basic education students (early childhood education, primary education, secondary education and youth and adult education) enrolled in public and philanthropic schools (MINISTÉRIO DA EDUCAÇÂO E CULTURA, 2009).

In the kindergartens in the municipality of Rio das Ostras, the menus are produced by qualified nutritionists from the Department of Education, the Nutrition Division (DINU) and passed on to the operating company. These menus are produced respecting "the food culture, the epidemiological profile of the population served and the agricultural vocation of the region" (BRASIL, 2009 b).

The menu in question is calculated to meet the nutritional needs of the students, following the criteria cited by Resolution/CD/FNDE No. 38, OF JULY 16, 2009, which states that when two or more meals are offered, they must meet at least, 30% of the daily nutritional needs of students enrolled in basic education, part-time, and at least 70% for students enrolled in basic education, including those located in indigenous communities and in areas remaining from quilombos, full-time.

The menus also respect the age groups and special needs of the students, as well as offering at least three portions of fruit and vegetables (200g/pupil/week), in compliance with interministerial ordinance 1010, which restricts the supply of foods high in fat, saturated fat, trans fat, free sugar and salt, thus valuing food as a strategy for promoting health, by resizing the actions developed in everyday school life (BRASIL, 2009 a; BRASIL, 2006).

At the beginning of 2014, when this research began, the city had four municipal nurseries.

Schools must serve all children enrolled in the school system free of charge

(BRASIL, 1996), and it is compulsory to offer a place in the public nursery school closest to the child's home from the day the child reaches the age of four (BRASIL, 2008).

The company contracted by Rio das Ostras City Hall to distribute meals to all public schools and nurseries in the municipality aims to meet the nutritional needs of students while they are at the institution, contributing to their development and learning, as well as promoting the formation of healthy habits.

Most of the children's meals, including the main meals, are eaten in the school environment, requiring greater care with quality, quantity and nutritional value. In this study, the menu offered was not surveyed, but it is worth highlighting the meals offered: breakfast, lunch, afternoon snack and dinner.

Throughout the school year, the company's nutritionists carry out training sessions with the cooks and caterers, nutritional education activities with the children and talks with parents, as well as taking part in the Health at School Week and Food Education Week events. In partnership with the Health at School Program, activities were carried out to encourage the consumption of fruit and vegetables.

6.1 Nutritional characteristics of preschoolers

Although it is dynamic and continuous, the growth process varies. This inconstancy tends to be reflected in the preschooler's diet, with periods of lower and higher food intake (BRASIL; DEVINCENZI & RIBEIRO, 2005, *apud* Silva & Mura, 2011, p. 409). As a professional working in situations where there is interaction between man and food, nutritionists must provide parents with appropriate guidance when growth slows down, promoting health in the school environment through educational and assistance activities (COSTA *et al*, 2001).

The pre-school period is marked, among other factors, by the acquisition of skills; however, during this phase, the speed of growth slows down, leading to a reduction in appetite (MANHAN; ESCOTT-STUMP, 2005). According to the authors, preschoolers are making discoveries and acquiring a certain degree of independence, which is why they begin to refuse foods that were previously easily accepted. This position is shared by Vitolo (2008), according to whom the discovery of objects and the child's lack of attention when walking are aspects that contribute to a lack of interest in food.

Studies have shown that preschoolers tend to develop an aversion to contact with new foods, often choosing those that belong to their dietary routine. This tendency reveals that preschoolers determine their eating patterns and, consequently, their preferences (RAMOS & STEIN, 2000).

Although these characteristics lead preschoolers to tend to be underweight, many studies have found that obesity and overweight occur. Therefore, while respecting children's preferences and nutritional needs, educators should encourage them to try a variety of foods, preferably dishes that attract their attention (BRASIL, 1998).

7. Results and discussion

7.1 The relationship between the genetic characteristics of the population and the nutritional status of children

This study assessed 101 children from a public nursery school in Rio das Ostras, RJ. At the time of the research, the institution had 109 children: of the students assessed, 56 (55.4%) were girls and 45 (44.6%) boys, with ages ranging from eight months to 48 months. The age group between two and less than five was the most prevalent, representing 64.4% of the population studied, as shown in Table 1. In terms of place of residence, all the children lived in urban areas, close to the nursery.

TABLE 1- Characterization of the children in terms of gender and age group attended by the Valdira Flausino Rodrigues Nursery School, Rio das Ostras, RJ, 2014.

Variables	N	%
Sex		
Female	56	55,4
Male	45	44,6
Age		
Between eight months and less two years	36	35,6
Between two years and less than five years	65	64,4

According to the Ministry of Health (2009), nutritional status (NS) is defined as the result of the balance between nutrient intake and energy expenditure to meet individual and collective nutritional needs, and is also an excellent indicator of quality of life (MELLO, 2002).

In order to ascertain whether or not a child's growth is deviating from the norm, whether due to illness or unfavorable conditions, the assessment of nutritional status is essential for monitoring the health of preschoolers, with the aim of establishing interventions by health professionals. Thus, in order to improve the quality of life of the population, with the aim of establishing a greater number of interventions early on, this procedure should be applied to as many individuals as possible (MELLO, 2002).

The data in Table 2 is associated with the children's nutritional status. According to Engstrom and Anjos (1996), mothers' level of education directly influences their children's nutritional status, since the transfer of maternal knowledge can be associated with various factors. Thus, in the case of a population generally classified as lay, the choice of food consumption is guided by aspects such as access to a diversity of foods and income level (MACIEL et. al, 2012). (FIGUEIREDO; JAIME and MONTEIRO, 2008) associated low schooling and a young population with low consumption of fruit and vegetables.

Unlike the results found by Felisbino-Mendes, Campos and Lana (2010) and Cagliari *et.al* (2009), in which it was found that the majority of mothers had studied for four or fewer years in formal education, and by Martino *et al.* (2010), which found that 45.2% of mothers had not completed elementary school, the results collected at the Valdira Flausino Rodrigues nursery school showed that 27.7% of carers had completed secondary school, 9.9% were illiterate and only 2% had completed higher education - as shown in table 2.

TABLE 2- Level of education of the children's guardians

RESPONSIBLE PERSON'S EDUCATION

	N	
Illiterate	10	9,9
First degree incomplete	27	26,7
Complete first degree	28	27,7
High school incomplete	13	12,9
Completed high school	28	27,7
Technical course	9	8,9
Higher education incomplete	4	4,0

Complete university degree	2	2,0
Total	101	100

In addition to the level of education of those responsible, other factors are related to the child's nutritional status, such as family income (MOLINA et al, 2010). Studies carried out in various regions of the country have shown that children are more prone to weight deficit and growth retardation in low-income families (VITOLO, 2008). Contrary to the findings of these studies, the data collected at the daycare center in question showed that although 96% of those interviewed had an average monthly family income of up to two minimum wages, using the minimum wage of R$724.00 in force in 2014 as a yardstick, 51% of the preschoolers were eutrophic.

GRAPH 1- Monthly wage income of all household members

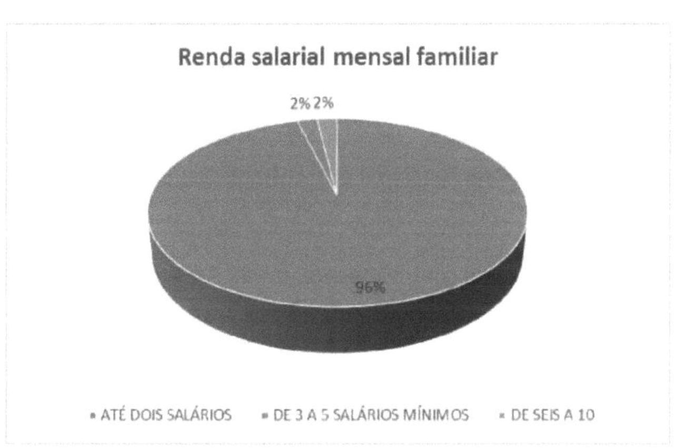

TABLE 3- Description of the mother's age, number of children and number of family income contributors.

MATERNAL AGE	n (%)
Less than 19	3(3)
Between 19 and 30	41(40,6)
31 or more	57(56,4)
NUMBER OF CHILDREN	
Only child	23(22,8)

More than one	78(77,2)
HOW MANY CONTRIBUTE TO	
FAMILY INCOME	
One	46(45,5)
Two	53(52,5)
Très a four	2(2)

Table 3 shows that 77.2% of mothers have more than one child and that 56.4% of them are aged 31 or over. Another significant figure relates to the number of people contributing to the family income: more than half of the population (52.5%) is made up of two people.

7.2 Factors that affect excess weight

Among the aspects that most contribute to the occurrence of overweight and obesity are environmental factors.

The media has contributed to the increase in cases of overweight. Research indicates that there is a direct relationship between cases of obesity and the number of hours spent watching television (Matsudo, Araùjo and Matsudo, 1998; Amaral and Palma, 2001). It can also be seen that the increase in time spent watching television has influenced eating habits, promoting a sedentary lifestyle (FERREIRA et al., 2012).

In this sense, a sedentary lifestyle also contributes to high obesity rates. This factor has occurred due to the technological and urban transformations that society has undergone (SPENCE; LEE, 2003). As a result, people's living conditions have changed, affecting family life habits and resulting in problems such as obesity (RIBEIRO, 2001).

In the Valdira Flausino Rodrigues nursery school, although the percentage of cases of eating in front of the television was relatively low (39.6%), the indices confirm the influence of the environment on the appearance of excess weight, highlighting the importance of systematizing physical activity, which prevents and combats obesity (Oliveira *et al*, 2003).

Another factor that contributes to overweight preschoolers is food advertising. Since children are the most likely to be affected by advertising, the media has a major influence on children's eating habits (MOURA, 2010). It is common to see advertisements for ultra-processed foods, with high concentrations of sugar, fat and salt. Recently, the Brazilian Institute for Consumer Protection evaluated the nutritional composition of thirty industrialized foods, the consumption of which is mainly aimed at children. In this research, IDEC showed that the levels of fat, sugar and salt present in "bolinhos" and "salgadinhos" were excessively higher than necessary for a balanced and healthy diet, and were therefore harmful to health (Monteiro and Castro, 2009). Therefore, the participation of parents in nutritional education projects can generate satisfactory results, thus influencing the home (MAHAN and ESCOTT-STUMP, 2002).

7.3 Assessment of children's nutritional status

The nutritional assessment of the children showed that 51% (n=52) of the preschoolers assessed were normal weight. On the other hand, 29% were at risk of being overweight, 13% were overweight and 6% were obese. Although the eutrophic rate in this study was significant, when added together, these percentages revealed worrying data, as 49% of the sample surveyed showed some alteration in their nutritional status and 19% were overweight or obese. There was also a low frequency of both thinness 1% (n=1) and marked thinness 0.0% (n=0).

GRAPH 2- Classification of nutritional status, according to BMI for age, of preschoolers at the Valdira Flausino Rodrigues Nursery School, Rio das Ostras, RJ, 2014.

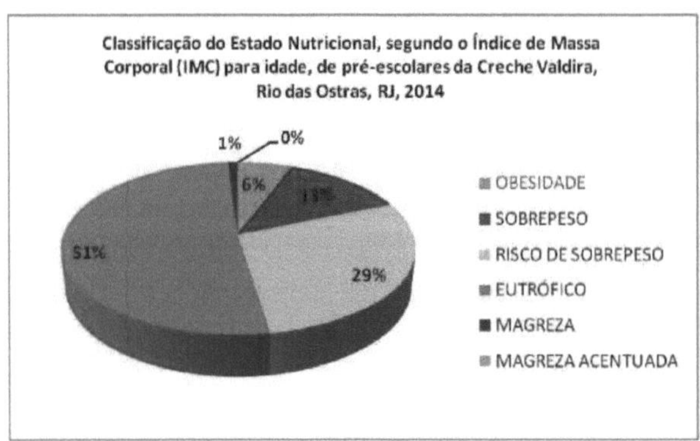

These results are similar to those found by Kuranishi *et al* (2001), whose research with pre-schoolers in Maringà - PR detected overweight in 13.02% of the children and obesity in 8.8%, resulting in 21.82% of overweight children.

Caciotori and Silva (2006) also found similar figures in a study carried out in the extreme south of Santa Catarina, where 25.76% of preschoolers were overweight.

In a study carried out in England, Brunded, Kitchiner and Buchan (2001) found that 14.7% of children were overweight and 5.4% were obese. These results show a trend towards an increase in overweight pre-school children.

In the 2006 National Demographic and Health Survey (PNDS), the prevalence of overweight among Brazilian children up to five years of age is 6.6%, reaching a higher proportion among those in the South region, at 8.8%, and a lower proportion in the North region, at 5.2% (PNDS, 2009).

When the children were stratified by gender, it was found that the number of girls showed a higher percentage of eutrophy: while they accounted for 58.9% (n=33) of the sample, the boys only accounted for 42.2% (n=19). The latter, however, had a higher prevalence of overweight risk (40%). Finally, the only case of thinness was detected in females.

TABLE 4 - Percentage classification of Nutritional Status, according to BMI for age, stratified by sex of the students at the Valdira Flausino municipal nursery school Rodrigues

IMC/AGE CLASSIFICATION	FEMALE	SEX	MALE	TOTAL
Eutrophic				
>Score-z -2 and <	33(58,9%)		19(42,2%)	52(51,5%)
Z-score +1				
Risk of				
Overweight				
>Escore-z +1 and	11(19,6%)		18(40%)	29(28,7%)
<Score-z +2				
Overweight				
> z-score +2 e<				
Z-score +3	8(14,3%)		5 (11,1%)	13(12,9%)
Obesity	3(5,36%)		3(6,67%)	6(5,9%)
> Z-score +3				
Thinness				
>Escore-z -3 e<	1(1,79%)		0	1(1%)
Score-z-2				
Accentuated thinness	0		0	0
< z-score-3				

TABLE 5: Classification of nutritional status according to the anthropometric index Height/Age, stratified by sex, of pupils at the Valdira Flausino Rodrigues municipal nursery school.

CLASSIFICATION HEIGHT/AGE	SEX		TOTAL(n)(%)
	FEMALE	MALE	
Very short stature for their age			
< z-score -3	1(1)	1(1)	2(2)
Short stature for age			
> z-score -3 and < z-score -2	1(1)	3(3)	4(4)
Age-appropriate height			
>Score-z -2	56(55,4)	39(38,6)	95(94)

Table 5 shows the results of the children's nutritional status, using the height-for-age index. It can be seen that the majority of them are eutrophic (n= 95) and that only four students had low height for age, three of whom were male and one female, and that two children were classified with the diagnosis of very low height, one of each sex. This result also showed that all children over the age of two had adequate height for their age.

Similar results were found by Mendonça (2009), who, when assessing two to five year old preschoolers attending public schools in Içara, Santa Catarina, found 98% to be eutrophic and only 2% with low height-for-age. In a study carried out in Rio Grande do Sul, with children in the same age group, Aires *et. al* (2011) found that all of them were adequate for the height-for-age index.

7.4 Children's food consumption

It is known that children's food consumption begins at birth. Since then, exclusive breast milk feeding has been encouraged, a nutritionally complete food that is essential for children's health in their first six months of life. It is a source rich in protective factors against infections and diseases common in infancy, and has no risk of contamination. It is also a sublime act, strengthening the bond of affection between mother and child (BRASIL, 2005 MS/PAHO, 2005).

Despite the many benefits of breastfeeding, several studies in Brazil have identified the early introduction of complementary foods, noting that a large number of children already have the habit of consuming various types of food by the age of six months (OLIVEIRA et al., 2005).

Using information from the SISVAN food consumption marker form, the frequency of food consumption was analyzed. The guardians of children aged between six months and less than two years were asked fifteen questions, nine of which related to the previous day's consumption, two about the last month, two about breastfeeding and two about the consumption of certain foods before the age of six months. For those with children aged between two and less than five years old, twelve questions were asked, six of which related to the previous day's consumption and six to food frequency.

TABLE 6 Period during which the child was exclusively breastfed

Period	Number of children	Percentage (%)
< 1 month	0	0
Up to 1 month	3	8
Up to 2 months	0	0
Up to 3 months	0	0
Up to 4 months	7	19
Up to 5 months	11	31
Up to 6 months	10	28
>6 months	5	14

Table 6 shows that only 28% of children were exclusively breastfed until they were six months old, a low rate for a practice that is proven to be important for the child's development. In a way, this practice corroborates the increase in the consumption of other milks, to the detriment of breast milk consumption (BRASIL, 2009).

Studies have shown that obesity can begin as early as the first year of life in predisposed individuals, a disease that arises from the combination of early weaning and the introduction of inadequate food (ESCRIVÂO *et al.*, 2000).

Still on the subject of the introduction of inappropriate foods before the age of six months, there was a high consumption of honey, molasses, sugar and sugary drinks: 77.8% said that they had introduced such foods into the child's usual diet and 58.3% also offered pot food or salty porridge before this age. Confirming the findings of Escrivao *et al* (2000), 22.2% of children aged between six months and less than two years were overweight or obese.

Therefore, the proper introduction of complementary foods presupposes the presence of foods from different groups: fruit, vegetables, cereals, legumes, meat and milk (BRASIL, 2014).

TABLE 7. previous day's food consumption of children between six months and less

than two years old

Food Consumption	N	%
Vegetables	24	66,7
Fruits	21	58,3
Meat (beef, chicken, fish, mii'ido. pig)	27	75
Beans	33	91,7
Pan food, no dinner	27	75

Table 7 shows the eating habits of children aged between six months and less than two years. In this age group, there was a significant consumption of vegetables (66.7%), fruit (58.3%) and beans (91.7%).

With regard to food frequency, the Ministry of Health recommends that at least three portions of fruit and three portions of vegetables should be consumed every day, with the importance of varying the consumption of these foods throughout the week (BRASIL, 2005).

Meat (beef, fish, chicken, pork and pork) was consumed the previous day by 75% of the children. This preparation should be included in the weekly menu, as it is known to be rich in protein and iron, a mineral with excellent bioavailability. Its deficiency is associated with iron deficiency anemia, delayed neuropsychomotor development and a decrease in the body's defenses and intellectual and motor capacity (BRASIL, 2005; PAHO, 2005).

Schaffazick's (2011) study of 62 children in Rio Grande do Sul found that the majority (77.3%) of the children ate pan food for dinner, a similar percentage to that found at the Valdira nursery school (75%).

TABLE 3- Consumption of soft drinks and industrialized juices or powdered soft drinks by children aged between six months and less than two years in the previous month

Food Consumption	n (%)
Soft drinks	19 (52,8)
Industrialized juice or powdered soft drink	29 (80,6)

When interviewed about their consumption of soft drinks in the previous month, those responsible reported that 52.8% of children had consumed this drink, in comparison with the 2nd Breastfeeding Prevalence Survey. This survey indicated that 4.9% of children aged between six and nine months had consumed soft drinks prior to data collection and that, considering the capitals and the Federal District as a whole, 11.6% of preschoolers aged between nine and twelve months had consumed soft drinks, a very high figure.

With regard to industrialized products (processed juice or powdered soft drinks), 80.6% of children consumed these products in the previous month.

In Brazil, data from the Family Budget Survey (2002-2003) showed that the purchase of sugar and soft drinks by Brazilian families comprised 13.4% of the energy value, while the percentage of fruit and vegetables corresponded to only 2.3%.

Some foods, such as soft drinks, snacks and processed juices, among others, have a high sodium content and should be discouraged (BRASIL, 2014).

TABLE 8. Consumption of cow's milk preparations on the previous day by children aged between six months and less than two years and between two years and less than five years.

Number of preparations	Children between six months and two years old (n=36)	Children between two and less than five years old (n=65)
	N (%)	N (%)
Not consumed	0(0)	5 (7,7)
Up to two preparations	23(**63,9**)	36 (**55,4**)
More than two preparations	13(36,1)	24 (36,9)

Table 8 shows the consumption of cow's milk by children aged between six months and less than two years and between two years and less than five years. It was observed that, in both age groups, the majority consumed up to two milk preparations a day.

Because it is a rich source of calcium, which is essential for the formation of teeth and bones, cow's milk is a recurring ingredient in children's diets. However, statistics reveal the early introduction of milk into the diets of preschoolers, reflecting a food culture that considers milk to be one of the most important foods for children's health (BRASIL, 2014).

In children between two and five years of age, dietary intake is directly related to their growth and development, a decisive and fundamental period in the formation of eating habits that tend to continue into adulthood; it is therefore important to encourage the consumption of a varied and balanced diet (COSTA et al., 2009).

According to the World Health Organization (2002), low consumption of fruit and vegetables is one of the main risk factors for obesity. These foods have important nutritional value for a healthy diet, as they are sources of micronutrients, fiber and nutrients with functional properties, such as carotenoids - yellow, green and/or red pigments found in vegetables - one of whose functions is to delay cellular aging. In addition, fruit and vegetables are low in calories in relation to the volume of food consumed, helping to maintain a healthy body weight (SONATI, 2009).

GRAPH 3- Average frequency of weekly food consumption in the two to under five age group reported by guardians. Rio das Ostras - RJ, 2014.

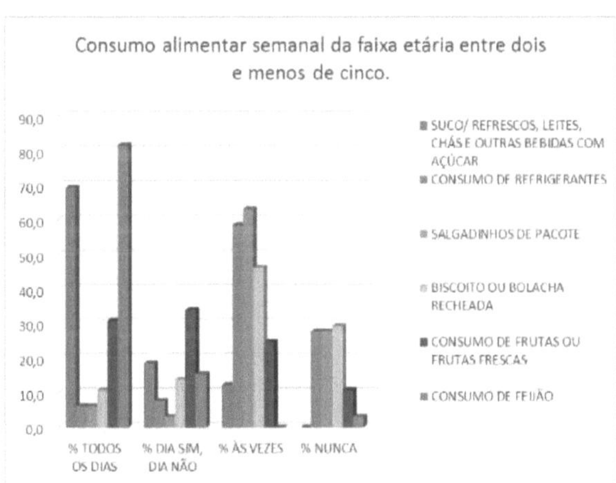

Graph 3 shows the frequency of weekly food consumption in the two to under five age group (n=65). It was found that the majority of children (69.2%) drink sugary drinks, such as juices, soft drinks, milk and tea sweetened with sugar, between five and seven times a week, the frequency indicated by the "every day" parameter. According to the World Health Organization (2004), excessive sugar consumption is associated with a higher risk of tooth decay, excess weight and other comorbidities. Although well accepted by the population, due to its pleasant taste and low cost, this food does not have many nutritional values, and is known for having empty calories, thus adding no nutritional value.

With regard to soft drink consumption, the "sometimes" parameter, corresponding to two or fewer times a week, was relevant. According to the study, 58.5% of children drink soft drinks on a weekly basis. On the other hand, only 6.2% drink this product every day.

This trend was also observed with regard to the consumption of filled cookies: while 46.2% of children consume them sporadically, i.e. two or fewer times a week, only 10.8% of them eat them five to seven days a week (the "every day" parameter). As for the consumption of packet snacks, only 6.2% eat them daily, while 63.1% eat them sometimes, which is alarming for the age group analyzed.

Although tastier and more pleasing to children's palates, these products are processed and contain a high calorie density. Furthermore, when eaten in excess, they can exceed the percentage of daily calories needed, leading to an increase in body weight (BRASIL, 2014).

Also according to graph 3, there was an average consumption of fruit or fruit juice: approximately 30.8% eat it every day and 33.8% every other day (three to four times a week). Next, the data shows that 81.5% of the children eat beans every day and only 3.1% (n=2) never eat this legume.

In general, the graph shows that milk consumption is adequate. As a result, there is a good intake of nutrients such as calcium, proteins, which are essential for bone growth, teeth and muscles (BRASIL, 2014). However, since drinks such as juices/refreshments, whether industrialized or not, are sweetened, it is likely that children are ingesting more sugar than recommended, which can lead to excess weight. These considerations were also found by Tuma *et al.* (2005). In their study, the early introduction of sugar into children's diets was observed: approximately 50% of the 230 preschoolers in nurseries in Brasilia used this food.

With regard to beans, the rates showed high consumption of this legume (81.5%), reflecting the region's food culture. Step 4 of Caderno de Atença Bàsica No. 38 indicates that this food should be eaten every day or at least five times a week, along with rice. On the other hand, the fruit/fresh fruit juice intake rates were average, indicating a proportional intake of vitamins and minerals.

Also according to the graph, there was a worrying consumption of packet snacks, filled cookies and soft drinks. Such eating habits are harmful to health, increasing the risk of chronic non-communicable diseases such as cardiovascular disease, diabetes mellitus, obesity, dyslipidemia and high blood pressure, since children consume high concentrations of salt, fat and sugar when they eat these treats. These foods should be eaten no more than twice a week, in small quantities (BRASIL, 2014; BRASIL, 2005).

TABLE 8. previous day's eating habits of children between two and less than five years old at Valdira Flausino Rodrigues nursery school, Rio das Ostras, RJ, 2014.

DIETARY PRACTICE	CHILDREN WHO CONSUMED	
	n =65	%
VEGETABLE CONSUMPTION	28	43,1
FRUIT CONSUMPTION	44	67,9
MEAT CONSUMPTION	53	81,5
TELEVISION CONSUMPTION	32	49,2
EATING PAN FOOD FOR DINNER	50	76,9
TOTAL	65	100

Table 8 shows the eating habits of children aged between two and less than five years old. A diet poor in fruit and vegetables and rich in industrialized foods has been a predictor of health problems, especially blood pressure levels (MOLINA, 2010).

Some researchers have warned that the availability of sugars has increased and the availability of fruit, vegetables and legumes has decreased in recent years in Brazil (SONATI, 2009).

Obesity Booklet No. 38 explains, in step 3 of the ten steps to a healthy diet for children between two and ten years old, that vegetables should be consumed daily, as part of the meal. Fruit can be distributed throughout the day at mealtimes, as it is rich in vitamins and minerals and improves the body's resistance.

The table shows that a high number of children ate meat the previous day (81.5%). It can also be seen that the majority of children (79.4%) eat pot food for dinner.

The prevalence of food consumption while watching television was relatively low (49.2%) in the study. Rossi et al. (2010), in a systematic review of the literature, revealed that the association between television and food consumption was evident in 85% of the articles and the association with obesity appeared in 60% of the articles. By identifying that time spent in front of the television is associated with inadequate eating habits and reduced physical activity, the habit of watching television is revealed as an important factor that can lead to obesity among children and adolescents.

The study carried out in nursery schools in the Federal District (DF) showed that the food consumption profile was high for dairy products, rice/meat, beans, sugar, bread and margarine; there was average consumption of fruit, vegetables, beef, chicken, eggs and cookies; low consumption of fish, offal, juices/cheeses and breast milk, as well as the early introduction of snacks, soft drinks, fast food, canned and sausage products and sweets. Thus, the occurrence of excess weight may reflect the dietary pattern of this population, indicating the need for education and health interventions to prevent chronic non-communicable diseases and improve quality of life (TUMA, COSTA and SCHMITZ, 2005).

8. Conclusion

The study under analysis reflects the process of food and nutritional transition taking place in Brazil, a trend also observed in the municipality of Rio das Ostras (RJ).

During the survey, a high percentage of overweight - obesity, overweight and risk of overweight - was observed in both age groups, as well as low levels of thinness and marked thinness, according to the BMI for Age. For the Height-for-Age index, a low percentage of short stature (and very short stature) was found, and this deviation was only observed in preschoolers aged six months to less than two years.

With regard to food consumption, good prevalence rates were found for the intake of vegetables, fruit, beans and meat in the age group between six months and less than two years. These rates demonstrate the diversification of these children's diets, preventing vitamin and mineral deficiencies. With regard to preschoolers between two and less than five years old, although meat consumption was significant, the intake of vegetables was relatively low. Both age groups, however, had significant levels of milk intake, with consumption of up to two preparations a day.

The majority of children between the ages of two and less than five have eaten sweets - packet snacks, cookies and soft drinks - two or fewer times a week. This consumption serves as a warning to society, because these foods are high in fat, salt and sugar and can lead to chronic diseases. The practice of eating while watching television was another negative aspect. Although this rate was relatively low, time in front of the television is related to inadequate eating habits and reduced physical activity, and in many cases is associated with obesity.

With regard to exclusive breastfeeding up to six months of age, low rates were found, in contrast to the consumption of soft drinks and industrialized juices, whose rates were significant, indicating early consumption of these drinks.

Knowing this information allows local managers and Family Health and School Health Program teams to implement strategies aimed at improving health conditions related to food and nutrition. It is therefore believed that the results obtained will serve as a warning to encourage the implementation of measures to help reduce cases of overweight and obesity in this community.

9. REFERENCES

ABRANTES, Marcelo M., LAMOUNIER, Joel A., COLOSIMO, enrico A. Prevalence of overweight and obesity in children and adolescents in the Southeast and Northeast regions. **Jornal de Pediatria** - Vol. 78, N°4, 2002.

AIRES, A. P. et al. Consumption of industrialized foods in preschoolers. **Revista da AMRIGS**, Porto Alegre, v., 55, n. 4, Oct./Dec. 2011.

AMARAL, A. P. de A. P.; PALMA, A. Epidemiological profile of obesity in children: relationship between television, physical activity and obesity. **Revista Brasileira Ciência e Movimento,** Brasilia, v. 9, n. 4, p. 19-24, 2001.

BIZZO MLG, Leder L. Nutritional education in the national curriculum parameters for elementary school. **Rev Nutr** 2005; 18:661-667.

BRASIL, 1996. **Guidelines and Bases Law**. Law No. 9.394/96, of December 20, 1996.

BRAZIL, 2005. Ministry of Health. **Food guide for children under 2** years **old/Ministry** of Health, Pan American Health Organization. - Brasilia: Editora do Ministério da Saùde, 2005.152 p.: il. - (Series A. Normas e Manuais Técnicos).

BRAZIL, 2009. Ministry of Health. Health Care Secretariat. Department of Primary Care. **Health at school** /Brasilia: Ministry of Health, 2009. 96 p. : il. - (Series B. Textos Bàsicos de Saùde) (Cadernos de Atença Bàsica ; n. 24)

Brazil, 2009. Ministry of Health. Health Care Secretariat. Department of Programmatic and Strategic Actions. **II Pesquisa de Prevalência de Aleitamento Materno nas Capitais Brasileiras e Distrito Federal/Ministério** da Saùde, Secretaria de Atença à Saù, Departamento de Açôes Programàticas e Estratégicas. - Brasilia: Editora do Ministério da Saùde, 2009. 108 p.: ill. - (Series C. Projects, Programs and Reports).

BRAZIL, 2011. Ministry of Health. Health Care Secretariat. Department of Primary Care. **Guidelines for the collection and analysis of anthropometric data in health services: Technical Standard for the Food and Nutrition Surveillance System -**

SISVAN / Ministry of Health, Secretariat for Health Care, Department of Primary Health Care. 76 p. : il. - (Series G. Estatistica e Informaçao em Saù).

BRAZIL, 2012. Ministry of Health. Health Care Secretariat. Department of Primary Care. **Child health: growth and development** - Brasilia: Ministério **da Saùde,** 2012. 272 p.: ill. - (Cadernos de Atença Bàsica, no. 33)

BRAZIL. Ministry of Health. Ministry of Planning, Budget and Management. Brazilian Institute of Geography and Statistics - IBGE. **Family Budget Surveys 2008-2009,** 2009.

Brazil. Ministry of Health. **National demographic and health survey of children and women - PNDS 2006: dimensions of the reproductive process and child health**. Brasilia, DF, 2009. 300 p. Available at:

http://bvsms.saude.gov.br/bvs/pnds/saude_nutricional.php

BRAZIL. Ministry of Health. **Protocols for the Food and Nutrition Surveillance System** - SISVAN in health care. Brasilia: Ministry of Health, 2008 (Series B. Textos Bàsicos de Saùde).

BRAZIL. Ministry of Health. Health Care Secretariat. Department of Primary Health Care. **National Food and Nutrition Policy** / Ministry **of** Health, Health Care Secretariat. Department of Primary Health Care. - 1. edition, 1. reprint - Brasilia: Ministry of Health, 2013. 84 p. : il.

BRAZIL. Ministry of Health. Health Care Secretariat. Department of Primary Care. **Strategies for the care of people with chronic illness: Obesity** / Ministry of Health, Secretariat of Health Care, Department of Primary Care. - Brasilia: Ministry of Health, 2014. 212p.:il.- (Cadernos da Atença Bàsica, n.38).

BUNDRED P, Kitchiner D, Buchan I. **Prevalence of overweight and obese children between 1989 and 1998: population based series of cross sectional** studies. BMJ [journal on the Internet]. 2001 [access on July 24, 2018]; 322: 326-28. Available at:

http://translate.google.com.br/translate?hl=ptBRsl=enu=ncbi.nlm.nih.gov/pub
med

CACIOTORI, P. F.; SILVA, L. S. M. **Prevalence of overweight and obesity in preschool children seen in 2005 at the clinical outpatient clinic of the University of the Extreme South of Santa Catarina. 2006.** Available at:

<http://200.18.15.7/medicina/tcc/ 2006_01/2006_01_ r47.pdf>. Acesso em : 18 nov. 2015.

CAGLIARI, Mayara Poliane Pires; PAIVA, Adriana Azevedo; QUEIROZ, Daiane; ARAÙJO, Emmanuele de Souza. Food consumption, anthropometry and morbidity in preschoolers from public day-care centers in Campina Grande, Paraiba. Nutrire: **Revista da Sociedade Brasileira de Alimentaçâo e Nutriçâo** = Journal Brazilian Society Food Nutrition, Sao Paulo, SP, v. 34, n. 1, p. 29-43, Apr., 2009.

COSTA, AGM; GONÇALVES AR, SUART DA, SUDA G, PIERNAS P, LOURENA LR et al. Evaluation of the influence of nutritional education on children's eating habits. **Rev Inst Ciênc Saùde**. 2009;27(3):237-43.

ENGSTROM, Elyne M. ; ANJOS, Luiz A. Relationship between maternal nutritional status and overweight in Brazilian children. **Rev. Saùde Pùblica**, 30 (3): 2339, 1996.

ESCRIVÂO, Maria Arlete M.S.; OLIVEIRA, Fernanda Luisa C. ; TADDEI, José Augusto de A.C. ; LOPEZ, Fàbio Ancona . Exogenous obesity in childhood and adolescence. **Jornal de Pediatria** - Vol. 76, Supl.3, 2000.

FELISBINO-MENDES, Mariana Santos; CAMPOS, Mirelle Dias; LANA, Francisco Carlos Félix. Evaluation of the nutritional status of children under the age of 10 in the municipality of Ferros, Minas Gerais. **Rev. esc. enferm.** USP, Sao Paulo, v. 44, n. 2, jun. 2010. Available at

Paulo, v. 44, n. 2, jun. 2010. Disponível em <http://www.scielo.br/scielo. php?script=sci_arttext&pid=S0080-234201000000003&lng=pt&nrm=iso>.

Accessed on March 12, 2015.

FERNANDES, Marcela de Melo, PENHA, Daniel Silva Gontijo, BRAGA, Francisco de Assis. Childhood obesity in public school children: prevalence and consequences for flexibility, explosive strength and speed, **Rev. Educ. Fis./UEM** v. 23, n. 4, p. 629-634, 4. Trim. 2012

FERREIRA, Marcos Santos; CASTIEL, Luis David and CARDOSO, Maria Helena Cabral de Almeida. **The pathologization of sedentary lifestyles**. Saùde soc.[online]. 2012, vol.21, n.4, pp.836-847.

FIGUEIREDO, Iramaia Campos Ribeiro; JAIME, Patricia Constante and MONTEIRO, Carlos Augusto. Factors associated with fruit and vegetable consumption in adults in the city of Sao Paulo. **Rev. Saùde Pùblica** [online]. 2008, vol.42, n.5, pp.777-785.

FILHO, Malaquias Batista, RISSIN, Anete. The nutritional transition in Brazil: regional and temporal trends. **Cad. Saùde Pùblica,** Rio de Janeiro, 19(Suppl. 1):S181-S191, 2003

GUIMARÂES, Lenir V., BARROS, Marilisa B.A. As diferenças de estado nutricional em pré-escolar de rede pubùblica e a transiçao nutricional. **Jornal de Pediatria** - Vol. 77, N°5, 2001. Available at :

http://bvsms.saude.gov.br/bvs/publicacoes/pesquisa_prevalencia_aleitamento_materno.pdf.

KURANISHI, L. T. et al. **Evaluation of the nutritional status of preschoolers enrolled in day-care centers in Maringà -PR in 2001. Maringà, 2001**. Available at:

http://www.saudebrasilnet.com.br/premios/saude/premio2/trabalhos/ 025.pdf.

Accessed: Nov. 18, 2015.

LOHMAN, T. G.; ROCHE, A. F. & MARTORELL, R., 1988. **Anthropometric**

Standardization Reference Manual. Champaign, Illinois: Human Kinetics.

MACIEL, E. S.; SONATI, J. G.; MODENEZE, D. M.; VASCONSELOS, J. S.; VILARTA, R.. Food intake, nutritional status and level of physical activity in a Brazilian university community. **Revista de Nutriçâo**, v. 25, n. 6, p 707718, 2012.

MAHAN, L. K, ESCOTT-STUMP, S. **Krause: Food, Nutrition and Diet Therapy.** 10ª edition. Ed. Roca, 2002.

MARTINO HS, FERREIRA AC, PEREIRA CN, SILVA RR. **Anthropometric evaluation and food intake of preschool children at municipal educational centers, in South of Minas Gerais State, Brazil.** Cienc Saude Colet. 2010;15:551-558.

MATSUDO, VKR; ARAÙJO, T. Level of physical activity in children and adolescents from different regions of development. **Rev. Bras. Ativ. Fis. Saùde.** 1998; 3(4); 14-26.

MELLO, E. D. O que significa a avaliaçao do estado nutricional. **Jornal de Pediatria,** Rio de Janeiro, v. 78, n. 5, 2002.

MENDONÇA, Andreia. **Evaluation of the nutritional status of preschoolers aged 2 to 5 attending public schools in the municipality of Içara/Santa Catarina.** Course Conclusion Paper. Criciùma, July 2009.

Ministry of Education and Culture. **National Education Guidelines and Bases Law.** Law No. 9.394/96, published in the DOU of December 23, 1996, Section I, p. 27839. Sao Paulo: Official State Press, 1996.

MOLINA et al. Socioeconomic predictors of children's diet quality. **Rev Saùde Pùblica, 2010**;44(5):785-92. Article available in Portuguese and English at:

www.scielo.br/rsp.

MONTEIRO, Carlos Augusto; CASTRO, Inês Rugani Ribeiro de. Why it is necessary to regulate food advertising. **Cienc. Cult.** [online]. 2009, vol.61, n.4, pp. 56-59. ISSN 2317-6660.

OLIVEIRA Ana Mayra A.; CERQUEIRA Eneida M.M; SOUZA, Josenira da Silva; OLIVEIRA, Antônio César. Childhood overweight and obesity: Influence of biological and environmental factors in Feira de Santana, BA. **Arq Bras Endocrinol Metab 2003**;vol.47, n.2, pp.144-150. ISSN 1677-9487.

OLIVEIRA, Cecilia, FISBERG L., Mauro. Obesity in Childhood and Adolescence - A Real Epidemic. **Arquivo Brasileiro Endocrinologia & Metabologia,** Sao Paulo, vol 47 n° 2 April 2003. Available at:

http://www.scielo.br/scielo.php?script=sci_arttext&pid=S00042730200300020 0001&lng=pt&nrm=iso>. Acesso em: 19 out. 2014.

OLIVEIRA, lucivalda P. Magalhaes de ; ASSIS, Ana Marlùcia O. ; GOMES, Gecynalda Soarès da Silva ; PRADO, Matildes da S. ; BARRETO, Mauricio L. . **Duration of breastfeeding, diet and associated factors according to living conditions in Salvador, Bahia, Brazil, 2005.**

PANPANICH, R, Garner P. **Growth monitoring in children**. Cochrane Database Syst Rev. 2000;(2):

POLLA, Simone Fàtima, SCHERER, Fernanda. Food and nutritional profile of schoolchildren in the municipal school system of a municipality in the interior of Rio Grande do Sul. **Caderno de Saùde Coletiva**, 2011, Rio de Janeiro, 19 (1): 111-6

RIBEIRO, I. C. **Obesity among public school children in Vila Mariana - São Paulo: a case-control study.** 2001. 115f Dissertation (Master's Degree in Nutrition). Paulista School of Medicine, University of Sao Paulo, Sao Paulo, 2001.

ROSSI, C. E. et al. Influence of television on food consumption and obesity in children and adolescents: a systematic review. **Rev. de Nutriçâo**, v. 23, n. 4, jul./ago.2010.

SCHAFFAZICK, Ana Luiza. **Nutritional status and food consumption of children registered in the Food and Nutrition Surveillance System of the municipality of Lagoa dos Très Cantos -RS, 2011**. Specialization in Public Health. Federal University of Rio Grande do Sul, Faculty of Medicine, Department of Social

Medicine. Porto Alegre, 2011.

SILVA, S. M. C. S. da; MURA, J. D. P. **Treatise on Food, Nutrition and Diet Therapy**. 2nd edition, ROCA, 2011.

SONATI, Jaqueline Girnos. School Feeding and Health. In: BOCCALETTO, E.M.A; MENDES, R.T. (eds.). **Food, activity**

physical activity and age of life of schoolchildren in the municipality of vinhedo/SP. Campinas: IPES Editorial, chap. 4. p. 31-33, 2009.

SPENCE, J. C.; LEE, R. E. **Toward a comprehensive model of physical activity**. Psychology of sport and exercise, Amsterdam, v. 4, p. 7-24, 2003.

TUMA, Rahilda Conceiçao Ferreira Brito; COSTA, Teresa Helena Macedo da; SCHMITZ, Bethsàida de Abreu Soares. Anthropometric and dietary assessment of preschoolers in three day-care centers in Brasilia, Distrito Federal. **Revista Brasileira Saùde Materno Infantil**, Recife, v. 5, n. 4, p. 419-428, Oct./Dec. 2005. Available at

<http://www.scielo.br/scielo.php?script=sci_arttext&pid=S1519382920050004 00005&lng=pt&nrm=iso>. Acesso em 15 fev . 2015

VITOLO, Màrcia Regina. Nutriçao: da gestação ao envelhecimento/ Nutrition from pregnancy to eldery.Rio de Janeiro; Ed. Rubio; 2008. 628 p. illustrated. Tab. Graph.

WHO (World Health organization, 1995. Physical status: The use and interpretation of anthropometry. Technical report series 834.Geneva: WHO).

10. ANNEXES

ANNEX 1. INFORMED CONSENT FORM

<table>
<tr><td>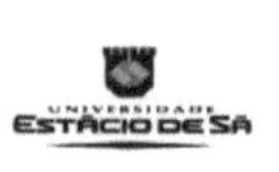</td><td>RESEARCH: Prevalence of overweight and its association with food consumption in children at a public kindergarten in the municipality of Rio das Ostras</td></tr>
</table>

This document will provide you with information and ask for your consent to take part in the research mentioned above, which will be carried out by the postgraduate course in Nutrition at the Estàcio de Sà University.

Please read the following information carefully before giving your consent.

RESEARCH PARTICIPANT IDENTIFICATION DATA

Name of Person in Charge: .... Sex

Gender: Male (   ) Female (....) Date of Birth: ..../ .... /

Address:

    Neighborhood

o:

City Phone ....: Ema

il:

Name of Student: ....Sex

o: ( ) M   ()   FDate of ....Birth: .... /........../

Research Protocol Title: xxxx Research Sub-Area: xxxxx

Lead researcher: Aline Valéria Martins Pereira.

Research risk assessment:

( ) Minimum Risk   ( ) Medium Risk   ( ) Low Risk (   ) Higher Risk

(x) No risk

Objectives and rationale: To investigate the prevalence of overweight and its association with food consumption in children at a public kindergarten in the municipality of Rio das Ostras - RJ.

This study is justified by the increase in the number of overweight children in Brazil and, above all, by the risks associated with this condition, such as greater vulnerability to the development of *diabetes mellitus*, dyslipidemia and hypertension, even in young people. In this way, the data to be investigated is extremely important for children and their guardians, as well as for health professionals in order to know the nutritional status of these children, as well as its association with food consumption. These results can facilitate the implementation of interventions that minimize the prevalence of overweight in these children and protect their health.

It should also be noted that, to date, there have been no studies evaluating the nutritional status of children enrolled in the Municipal Nurseries of Rio das Ostras - RJ.

Your participation in this survey includes the following procedures:

a) Answer a questionnaire on food consumption frequency and an interview on family eating habits;

b) Allows you to measure students' weight and height;

Risks and inconveniences: No risks

Potential benefits: xxxxx

If you have any considerations or questions about the ethics of the research, you can contact the Research Ethics Committee (CEP) of the Estácio de Sá University, during business hours, by e-mail at cep.unesa@estacio.br or by telephone at (21) 3231-6139. For this research, there will be no cost to the participant at any stage of the study. Likewise, there will be no financial compensation related to your participation. You will have full and complete freedom to refuse to participate or to withdraw your consent at any stage of the research.

I believe that I have been sufficiently informed about the information I have read or that has been read to me, describing the study: Prevalence of overweight and its association with food consumption in children of a public nursery school in the Municipality of Rio das Ostras.

The purposes of this research are clear. Likewise, I am aware of the procedures to be carried out, their discomforts and risks, the guarantees of confidentiality and ongoing clarification. It is also clear that my participation is free of charge. I voluntarily agree to take part, knowing that I can withdraw my consent at any time, before or during the procedure, without penalty or prejudice.

This form will be signed in two (2) copies of equal content, one for the research participant and one for the person responsible for the research.

ANNEX2 . SOCIO-ECONOMIC QUESTIONNAIRE FOR PARE

RESPONSIBLE

Full name: ____

Age: Do you have any other children?

What is your marital status?

( ) Single

( ) Married

( ) Widowed

( ) Other

What is your level of education?

( ) Illiterate

( ) Primary school incomplete

( ) Complete primary school

( ) Secondary school incomplete

( ) High school completed

( ) Technical course

( ) Incomplete university degree

( ) Higher education completed

Who do you currently live with?

( ) With parents and/or other relatives.

( ) With spouse and/or child(ren).

( ) With friends (sharing expenses or as a favor).

( ) Alone.

How many people live in your house (including you)?

( ) Two.

( ) Three.

( ) Four.

( ) Five.

( ) More than 6.

( ) I live alone

How many people contribute to your family's income?

( ) One.

( ) Two.

( ) Three to four.

( ) Five to six.

( ) More than six.

What is your monthly family income? (Consider the sum of the incomes of everyone in your household) (Minimum wage = R$ 724.00)

( ) up to two minimum wages.

( ) from three to five minimum wages.

( ) from six to 10 minimum wages.

( ) more than 10 minimum wages.

ANNEX 3. REFERENCE AND COUNTER-REFERENCE FORM ADAPTED FOR THE SCHOOL HEALTH PROGRAM.

ESTADO DO RIO DE JANEIRO
MUNICÍPIO DE RIO DAS OSTRAS

FICHA DE REFERÊNCIA E CONTRA- REFERENCIA

O Programa Saúde na Escola (PSE) esteve na 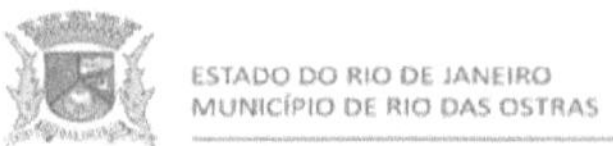 Creche Valdira Flausino Rodrigues realizando **Avaliação Nutricional**. Os educandos foram pesados e medidos e os dados obtidos foram analisados conforme recomendação do Ministério da Saúde para avaliação populacional.

O aluno_______________________________________ apresentou peso de _______ kg e altura de ________ m, sendo classificado (a) com _________________. Gostaríamos de esclarecer que para o diagnóstico nutricional individual, outros métodos de avaliação podem e devem ser realizados, firmando um parecer mais conclusivo.

Sendo assim, faz-se necessário que o (a) senhor (a) leve (a) a unidade básica de saúde (UBS) para uma avaliação mais detalhada e acompanhamento/tratamento.

Portanto, encaminhamos ___________________________________, para acompanhamento nutricional no Posto de Saúde do ______________________________.

____
Assinatura do Responsável

SECRETARIA DE EDUCAÇÃO
Rua Guanabara, 3603 - Extensão do Bosque
Rio das Ostras - RJ - CEP: 28893-158

SECRETARIA DE SAÚDE
Rua Jandira Morais Pimentel, 504 - Centro
Rio das Ostras - RJ - Brasil - CEP: 28893-046

PREFEITURA
RIO DAS
OSTRAS

www.riodasostras.rj.gov.br

ANNEX 4. SISVAN FOOD FREQUENCY QUESTIONNAIRE (QFA)

	Ministério da Saúde/ SAS/ DAB/ CGPAN SISTEMA DE VIGILÂNCIA ALIMENTAR E NUTRICIONAL	
	Estabelecimento de Saúde	Nº CNES*
	Nome ou Matrícula do Profissional de Saúde	

Nome completo*	Data de nascimento:* / /
Endereço completo*	
Documentação (tipo, número e outras especificações)	Data de preenchimento:* / /

* Campos de preenchimento obrigatório (fundo cinza).

CRIANÇAS MENORES DE 6 MESES

1. A criança **ontem** mamou leite do peito? ☐ Sim (pule para a pergunta 3) ☐ Não

2. **Se não**, até que idade seu filho mamou no peito? ☐ Nunca ___ meses **OU** ___ dias

3. Até que idade seu filho ficou em aleitamento materno exclusivo?
(ler para o entrevistado: **aleitamento exclusivo é só leite do peito, sem chá, água, leites, outras bebidas ou alimentos**)
☐ <1 mês ou nunca ☐ até 1 mês ☐ até 2 meses ☐ até 3 meses ☐ até 4 meses ☐ até 5 meses ☐ Ainda está em aleitamento materno exclusivo

4. A criança **ontem** recebeu (ler as alternativas para o entrevistado - pode marcar mais de uma alternativa): ☐ Leite do peito ☐ Chá/Água ☐ Leite de vaca ☐ Fórmula Infantil ☐ Suco de fruta ☐ Fruta ☐ Papa Salgada ☐ Outros

CRIANÇAS COM IDADE ENTRE 6 MESES E MENOS DE 2 ANOS

1. A criança **ontem** recebeu leite do peito? ☐ Sim (pule para a pergunta 3) ☐ Não

2. **Se não**, até que idade seu filho mamou no peito? ☐ Nunca ___ meses **OU** ___ dias

3. Até que idade seu filho ficou em aleitamento materno exclusivo?
(ler para o entrevistado: **aleitamento exclusivo é só leite do peito, sem chá, água, leites, outras bebidas ou alimentos**)
☐ <1 mês ou nunca ☐ até 1 mês ☐ até 2 meses ☐ até 3 meses ☐ até 4 meses
☐ até 5 meses ☐ até 6 meses ☐ > 6 meses ☐ Ainda está em aleitamento materno exclusivo

4. Ontem, quantas preparações (copos/mamadeiras) de leite a criança tomou? (qualquer tipo de leite animal: pó/fluido)
☐ Não tomou ☐ Até 2 (copos/mamadeiras) ☐ Mais que 2 (copos/mamadeiras)

5. **Ontem**, a criança comeu verduras/legumes (não considerar os utilizados como temperos, nem batata, mandioca, cará e inhame)? ☐ Sim ☐ Não

6. **Ontem**, a criança comeu fruta? ☐ Sim ☐ Não

7. **Ontem**, a criança comeu carne (boi, frango, porco, peixe, miúdos ou outras)? ☐ Sim ☐ Não

8. **Ontem**, a criança comeu feijão? ☐ Sim ☐ Não

9. **Ontem**, a criança comeu assistindo televisão? ☐ Sim ☐ Não

10. **Ontem**, a criança comeu comida de panela (comida da casa, comida da família) no jantar? ☐ Sim ☐ Não

11. A criança recebeu mel/melado/açúcar/rapadura **antes de 6 meses de idade**, consumido com outros alimentos ou utilizado para adoçar líquidos e preparações? ☐ Sim ☐ Não

12. A criança recebeu papa salgada/comida de panela (comida da casa, comida da família) **antes de 6 meses de idade**? ☐ Sim ☐ Não

13. A criança tomou suco industrializado ou refresco em pó (de saquinho) **no último mês**? ☐ Sim ☐ Não

14. A criança tomou refrigerante **no último mês**? ☐ Sim ☐ Não

15. A criança tomou mingau com leite ou leite engrossado com farinha ontem? ☐ Sim ☐ Não

CRIANÇAS COM IDADE ENTRE 2 ANOS E MENOS DE 5 ANOS

1. **Ontem**, quantas preparações (copos/mamadeiras) de leite a criança tomou? (qualquer tipo de leite animal: pó/fluido)
☐ Não tomou ☐ Até 2 (copos/mamadeiras) ☐ Mais que 2 (copos/mamadeiras)

2. **Ontem**, a criança comeu verduras/legumes (não considerar os utilizados como temperos, nem batata, mandioca, cará e inhame)? ☐ Sim ☐ Não

3. **Ontem**, a criança comeu fruta? ☐ Sim ☐ Não

4. **Ontem**, a criança comeu carne (boi, frango, porco, peixe, miúdos ou outras)? ☐ Sim ☐ Não

5. **Ontem**, a criança comeu assistindo televisão? ☐ Sim ☐ Não

6. **Ontem**, a criança comeu comida de panela (comida da casa, comida da família) no jantar? ☐ Sim ☐ Não

7. Com que frequência a criança toma sucos/refrescos, leites, chás e outras bebidas com açúcar/rapadura/mel/melado? (ler as alternativas para o responsável) ☐ Todos os dias (5 a 7x semana) ☐ Dia sim, dia não (3 a 4x semana) ☐ Às vezes (2 x semana ou menos) ☐ Nunca

8. Com que frequência a criança toma refrigerantes? (ler as alternativas para o responsável)
☐ Todos os dias (5 a 7x semana) ☐ Dia sim, dia não (3 a 4x semana) ☐ Às vezes (2 x semana ou menos) ☐ Nunca

9. Com que frequência a criança come salgadinho de pacote (aqueles industrializados feitos para crianças)? (ler as alternativas para o responsável) ☐ Todos os dias (5 a 7x semana) ☐ Dia sim, dia não (3 a 4x semana) ☐ Às vezes (2 x semana ou menos) ☐ Nunca

10. Com que frequência a criança come biscoito ou bolacha recheados? (ler as alternativas para o responsável)
☐ Todos os dias (5 a 7x semana) ☐ Dia sim, dia não (3 a 4x semana) ☐ Às vezes (2 x semana ou menos) ☐ Nunca

11. Com que frequência a criança come frutas ou bebe suco de frutas frescas? (ler as alternativas para o responsável)
☐ Todos os dias (5 a 7x semana) ☐ Dia sim, dia não (3 a 4x semana) ☐ Às vezes (2 x semana ou menos) ☐ Nunca

12. Com que frequência a criança come feijão? (ler as alternativas para o responsável)
☐ Todos os dias (5 a 7x semana) ☐ Dia sim, dia não (3 a 4x semana) ☐ Às vezes (2 x semana ou menos) ☐ Nunca

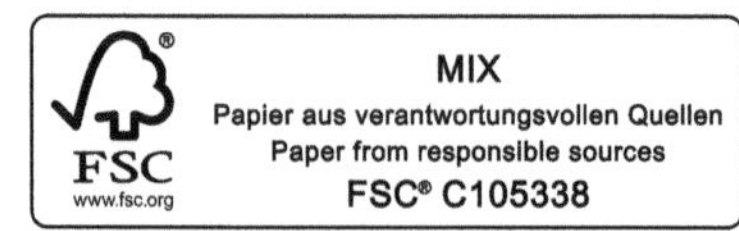

Printed by Books on Demand GmbH, Norderstedt / Germany